CARE LESS, LIVE MORE

How to Stop Giving a *You know what!*

By Oyam Zeza

TABLE OF CONTENTS

INTRODUCTION

∞

In life, there are many things that you do because you feel obliged to do them. Think about it. In some way, most of our lives revolve around trying to please someone, be it our boss, parents or friends. But, does it have to? How much do we have to give up, to make the people around us happy? To make ourselves happy?

To live happily, you have to realize that your happiness needs to be dependent on your actions and not on how others perceive you. You have to start caring less and living more. You have to stop giving a *you know what* about most things in life.

Take a minute to think about the following questions: Why do you live in this city? Why are you at your current job? Why do you care so much about what others feel? If your answer to any of the above questions was anything other than, 'Because I want to,' then this book is for you. It's time that you stopped caring about what others think and more about how you need to better yourself.

This book aims to help you to understand that caring less is sometimes beneficial rather than detrimental. Thank you for choosing this book, and I hope you enjoy it.

CHAPTER 1:

SAVE YOUR SANITY
AND YOUR LIFE

∞

It's only natural to care about what others think. We live in a world where sometimes, meeting society's expectations is the main priority because we are tuned to believe that the opinions of other people matter. Everybody can think of at least a dozen reasons why they have worried too much about what other people think.

How many times have you done something embarrassing? How often have you wondered *what are people going to think*? How many times have you stopped yourself from buying an outfit because it was loud or not in fashion and you worried about how people would react if you wore it? Have you ever made a career choice based on what your family thought was best for you? How many dates or engagements have you had to cancel because you were working overtime to please your boss? How many baby showers have you attended because you were worried that your friend might hate you if you didn't make it?

There are times in life when it seems that the worst that could happen to us is that somebody doesn't like us. As a result, you spend all of our efforts trying to please someone who may not even be thinking about you. People are always going to talk, and you need to accept that that us human nature. It is easy to get lost in being too concerned about what other people think, but you must not allow that to get the best of you. You lose focus in your own life by flooding your life with thoughts based upon what other people think, which is not healthy. In order to live a happy life, you need to stop caring about trivial things like the thoughts of some random person who has absolutely no power to impose his/her opinion on your life—and quite frankly, whose opinion does not matter! The truth is that people with strong opinions about the lives of others' are missing something in their own lives.

Another thing you need to be aware of is that there is a difference between being carefree and not caring at all. You should train yourself to care about the significant things in life without being bogged down by the nonsense. Much of what you see as problematic is as a direct result of your thought processes, and you need to look beyond the trivia and see the whole picture.

Believe it or not, the world isn't going to end if you take a day off from work or if you fail to live up to someone's expectations, your participation in events isn't do-or-die, and you are not responsible for cleaning up everyone else's mess. Events and meetings will happen with or without you. So, prioritize and care about the things that matter and don't spend all of your energy on every single insignificant event. You don't have to help organize everybody's birthday parties, baby showers, prom parties, etc.

You also don't need to make it your mission to make yourself likable by every person on this planet—it is an exhausting and entirely unnecessary job. The list of people to keep happy goes on into infinity and the saddest part is that the person who should be on that list is probably not even in it, and that person is YOU!

The bottom line is that no matter how much you try, there will always be people who are not pleased with you. You will either be too helpful or too unhelpful, too clingy, too aloof, too nice, or too mean. The list goes on and on. It's time to realize that you can never please everyone and that's OK. Once you realize and accept this, you will see that there are a bunch of people who care for you just as much as you care for them without you having to bend over backwards to please them. These are the people who matter. Everybody and everything else is dispensable. Once you learn to care less about everybody else and focus on these people and yourself, you will see how much less stressful your life is.

CHAPTER 2:

THE TRUTH ABOUT LIFE

∞

Let's talk about some things that most of us need to hear about life and the people around us. It's time to stop giving a flying *you know what,* and here's why:

People judge you all the time

What you must acknowledge and accept is the fact that people will always judge. Right now, there is probably someone judging you for the way you dress, or perhaps you are too loud, or too quiet! There is nothing you can do about this. No amount of flattery or rubbing shoulders with them is going to stop them from judging you. You know what would be great? If you stop caring about the judgement that others pass on you. The more you care about their judgment, the more fun they have judging you.

You don't need everybody's seal of approval

This might come as a shocker to most of you. But, embrace it. This is the truth. Everybody judges you, but what's even more shocking is that even if they do, it DOES NOT MATTER. When people don't like or disapprove of what you do, nothing changes in the universe; the world doesn't end, you don't die; life goes on. The more you ignore judgmental people, the better off you are. Worrying about judgmental people only wastes valuable time and resources.

Let's suppose that you changed your appearance to make people like you. Would that change really make you feel better? Would it give you a better life? Probably not. So, why waste your precious time caring?

Not giving a second thought to others is what makes your life better. It's time you embraced and lived this truth.

Find your people. They matter.

By this point in the book, you should realize that there are people who are bent on disliking or judging you, and that those people really should not matter. At this point, we are going to focus on the people that *do* matter. Ironically, these are the people we tend to ignore the most.

Relationships can be weird; be it with your family, or friends. These are the people with whom we have the strongest bonds, but these are also the people whom we take for granted. We may even ignore them in favor for strangers. We spend more time pleasing our bosses and neighbors but forget about our loved ones. Once we successfully impress someone, we then push them into the 'taken for granted' zone and move on the next stranger who we think we need to please.

However, the people we take for granted are the people we should cherish and keep closest to us because they like us for who we are—faults and all. We don't have to change ourselves to impress them. They make us feel safe and happy. We should stop focusing on others and make these people the center of our attention.

It all starts and ends with you.

The whole concept of caring less has nothing to do with the people around you. Rather, it has everything to do with you. If you choose to live your life based on your own standards and expectations, rather than trying to meet that of others', then you will live a life of much less stress. Sometimes we feel like saying *to hell with it all!* but we stop ourselves. There are times when you must allow yourself to get past that checkpoint.

Everyone has an 'internal eye', which is the part of your mind that is mindful of what you as an individual, consider unacceptable behavior. What is defined as acceptable and unacceptable varies from person to person and if you are always worried about what others think, then your internal eye will also begin to focus on instances when your behavior doesn't fit social norms. This when you subconsciously prevent yourself from doing things you would like to do. It can be something as simple as a body movement, to an entire change in personality. If you feel that wearing a dress makes people stare, then whenever you pick out clothes your internal eye will subconsciously prevent you from picking out that dress. This eye isn't you. It's what you think others want to see in you. It boxes you in. The good thing is, you can control it and prevent it from boxing you in. You are free to be yourself.

CHAPTER 3

HOW TO STOP CARING LESS AND LIVING MORE

∞

We are here, in this world, for a few decades. Don't lose yourself to other people's opinions and thoughts. Don't let yourself become a passive bystander in your own life. Here are some ways to stop giving a *you know what* and to start succeeding in life.

Look at yourself

No one knows you better than you do. To figure out what you care about, you first need to understand what you value. What you value is what is most important. Let your values guide you into making decisions. If you think you should teach kids in your spare time, then go ahead and do it. If you think you should adopt a dog, then adopt one despite what others might say. If you think you are good at organizing things, take charge of administrative work at the office. Take charge of your life in its entirety!

Do you want to sit in meetings every day? No? Then show your boss that you are more productive without these meetings.

Forget about being perfect

We have it drilled into our heads that we need to be perfect; that anything short of perfect is unacceptable. We always look for faults in ourselves and hold ourselves up against the highest mark we possibly can. Once you aim for perfection, you fall short, and your self-confidence takes a major hit. Why do we fall short? Because there is no way to be perfect. We are human. We can never be perfect. To reduce your burden, you need to let go of this need to achieve perfection.

Make the word 'no' a frequent word in your vocabulary

Caring about what people think can be dangerous because it can turn you into a people pleaser. The moment you start accommodating other individuals' in the hope that they will stop judging you, you have crossed a dangerous line because you eventually lose your ability to say no to people. You need to nip this in the bud before it becomes a habit. Learn how to say NO.

When you start caring less about the things that don't matter to you, you start viewing the world through a different pair of eyes. Caring less also means turning down more invitations to events you would rather not attend. This can be anything from baby showers to professional projects.

There are many instances where you need to step up and say *no*. Here are a few examples:

- Text messages from people who need your help on trivial tasks.

- Projects that make you put in more work than you should.

- A colleague trying to pawn off their work on to you by giving some lame excuse.

Sometimes these distractions can be a genuine cry for help, but most of the time they are just distractions.

Saying *no* in a professional environment can be hard because you don't want to get fired or offend a colleague. Simply find a way to say *no* without being rude: be respectful and professional. When start out saying *no*, you can offer an excuse or suggest an alternative, if it helps (but you are in no way obligated to do this). Nine times out of ten, people will agree with your alternative—ten times out of ten, life goes on. The easiest way to get out of things is to tell people that you have a lot of work and can't give your full attention to their work. This is a way to tell them no without being rude.

Don't let a negative opinion define who you are

Keep an open mind and don't let someone's negative opinion of you define you as a person. If for example, someone who barely knows you says you have anger issues, then don't take it to heart. They have hardly interacted with you to actually know you. Your close friends or family who have a better idea of your personality or character may have an opinion or two that you may not like. Still, you don't have to take it in a negative way. You can use it as an opportunity to improve yourself.

Most of you may already be stuck in that rut where you find it impossible to stop caring and reclaim your self-respect. It is never too late; you just need to be willing to lose a little and accept a few facts about life. Here are eight steps on how to gain control of your life:

Step 1: Understand why it doesn't matter

The very first step is to figure out why you are doing something. Why doesn't it matter what others think of you? Why should you care less?

Consider, if you are so worried about what other people think, then isn't it probable that other people are also concerned about how people perceive them? So, people are probably too busy worried about what others think about them to think about you.

Also, even if they are thinking about you, it should not bother you. What goes on in their heads is none of your concern because you can't control it. Whatever you can't control, you can't get rid of. So, focus on the things you can control, and stop caring about the rest.

Also, the good feeling you get after someone 'approves' of you, isn't going to last very long. As soon as you stop feeling that 'high' you will look for another person to seek approval from and so on. It's an endless cycle. Getting support feels good but it cannot drive you. It lasts for a short time. And then you'll be back to hating your life. The only way you can feel that 'high' all the time is if you approve of yourself. Do the things you want to do, when you want and where you want.

Step 2: Do things that embarrass you

Wear mismatched clothes; wear the loudest tie you can find. Wear flip-flops with a suit. Yes, I know you will look like a crazy person. That's the point. We are so worried about people laughing at us or mocking us. Wear your weird outfits and go to the busiest part of the city. Just observe how many people even look at you twice. You'll may be surprised that not even 50% of the people will notice your existence. Even the ones who see your outfit may just look at you, carry on, and forget about you in seconds.

What do you achieve by doing this? Well, for starters, you should realize that nobody will stop to gape at you (and if they do…so what?). Secondly, you should not feel bad. Initially, you may feel shy and awkward, but the more time you spend in your weird outfit, the more comfortable you become.

That was just one example. I encourage you to identify your mental blockades: find out that *you think* you can and can't do. Slowly, conquer them, one by one and treat society the same way.

Step 3: Accept yourself for who you are

Accept the fact that you are yourself and that there are parts of you that can't be changed. Accept that you can have your share of awkward moments. Don't try to avoid them.

Make a list of characteristics that you like about yourself and another list of the things you don't like. Try to improve the features that you don't like. You can even ask your friends and family to add to your list and help you develop. This will help build self-confidence.

Step 4: Refuse to be boxed in

People around you might try to limit your choices; put you in a box. But there are no boxes in life. Don't let anybody tell you otherwise.

Take the path you want to take. People might try to force you to choose between options they find acceptable, but don't let them dictate your ways. You don't have to choose between two good things. You can have both. Do you want a stellar professional career and a satisfying personal life? Do people tell you that it's near impossible? Don't listen to them. Give it a shot. You might be able to achieve what they deem impossible because *they failed.* You never know unless you try.

Live your life the way you want to. Don't live somebody else's by allowing them to box you in.

Step 5: Visualize success not failure

Instead of focusing on how you failed at something and the resulting embarrassment, focus on all the times when you succeeded. You can break down your goals into small parts. Once you have your parts, visualize yourself succeeding at each part.

For example, if you are embarrassed by how you speak in front of a crowd, then start by making small goals to overcome your fear. First, start talking at team meetings or in front of friends. Build up your confidence in stages. Once you conquer each stage of your goal, move on to the next.

Step 6: Surround yourself with confident people

Surround yourself with people who live their life by not caring about the world. Their lifestyle will rub off on you.

I have a friend, Brandon who is a great influence. He voices his opinions when he wants to, irrespective of whether it is the popular opinion or not. After observing him for a while, I realized that he was just voicing opinions that others were too scared to talk about.

Step 7: Be truthful

Are you one of those people who try to please everyone by not taking a side in an argument or discussion? This would be okay if it were just a discussion. But if you plan to avoid telling the truth because you want to please everybody, that isn't going to work for you. Nobody intends to work with or under somebody who can't stand up for themselves and tell the truth.

You need to call the nonsense if you see it. You don't have to be aggressive about it, but you can at least add your two cents worth when the topic or issue comes up.

However, you don't have to add any extra furnishings to the truth. Tell only your truth and not the truth you think others want to hear because, that would be—well a lie! This will help you come to terms with the fact that you don't have to please everyone. You will realize that telling the truth will make you more respected.

Step 8: Showcase the new you

Once you accomplish the previous seven steps, you should be ready to start your new life. You can now start exploring a whole world of opportunities that you previously closed because you cared too much about what people thought of you.

Do you want to start a new career? Go ahead. Just understand the consequences of starting again. Do you want to adopt a dog? Just make sure you prepare yourself for the responsibility of having a pet that depends on you.

Once you start walking down this path of discovery, you begin to realize that everyone who matters understands the choices you make. The ones who don't understand are the people who never mattered. In fact, people might respect you for choosing to direct your destiny instead of bowing to the pressure of society. This will only give you the confidence to unburden your stress and take over your world.

Start developing habits that are right for you. I don't mean habits like making your bed or brushing your teeth twice a day. No, I mean practices that let you live your life to the fullest. If you want to get fit, go to the gym regularly. If you want to feel calm, practice yoga. Do things that make you happy. Play basketball, maintain a blog and travel around the world. When you have things that make you happy, all adverse things in life become insignificant.

Learn to set goals that you care about. Forget about what other people want you to do. Set goals to accomplish your purpose, not the goals that accomplish that of others. Your aspirations and ambitions should come ahead of those of others. Don't give others any room to redirect your life goals. The easiest way to do this is by setting short term goals. When you set goals for the near future, they will be focused on your current aspirations. People will try to pressurize you into following the path they think is right for you. However, by focusing on short-term goals, you have your finish line in sight. This prevents you from getting deviated by all this pressure.

Please understand that none of these life changing experiences can happen if you don't take the first step and start caring less. It can only happen if you consciously adopt the changes and go out of your way to care less. You need to find the courage and determination to stop giving a *you know what* and do exactly what you want to do. That's the bottom line.

CONCLUSION

When you learn to start caring for the things that matter and stop caring for the millions of irrelevant things in life, you will live a whole new life. You will start to care less, and be less stressful. You will tell the entire world to get lost and live exactly how you want. So, be the person who takes control of their life!

It takes some practice to be able to shake off the reins that society and people have on you. But once you do, you'll see the world through new eyes. Making those changes might sound easy on paper, but nothing in life comes easy. If you want to stop giving a, *you know what*, then you better start taking your first steps in that direction. The stress-free life will be worth all the steps you need to take now.

I hope this book gave you enough courage to turn your world around by caring just enough. Thank you once again for choosing this book and good luck!

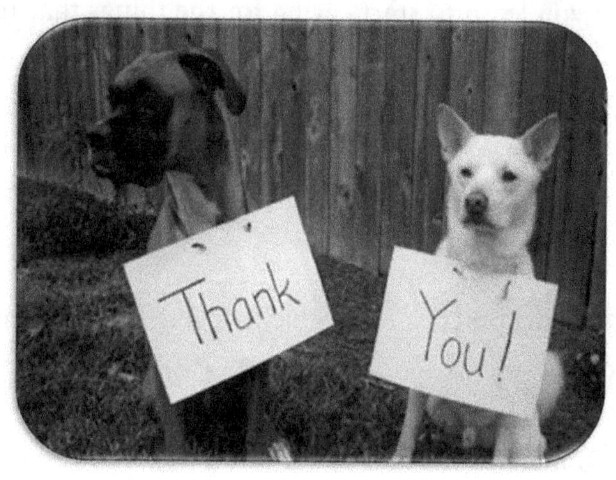

Finally, if you enjoyed this book, then I'd like to ask you for a favor. Will you be kind enough to leave a review for this book on Amazon? It would be greatly appreciated!

Thank you and good luck!

Check Out My Other Books

Below you'll find another one of my popular books that. Simply search for the title on the Amazon website or click on the title!

DASH Diet Made Easy: 25 DASH Diet Recipes for Beginners!

Diabetic Smoothie Recipes: 35 Easy & Delicious Smoothie Recipes for Diabetics